A Proposed Psychophysical Exercise and Treatment Regimen for Epilepsy

Epilepsy Treatment by Therapeutic Aromatic Penetration and Olfactory Intervention (ETTAPOI)

Author: Arghya Ray

Date: January 2016

Preface

Epilepsy is basically a disease of brain. There are certain varieties of this disease. Treatment of the disease is mainly based on chemotherapeutic interventions. Usage of artificially manufactured medicines and stimulators may create chronic to severe problems in the patients at a later stage. In fact, every allopathic medicine is known to have at least some minimal side effects that can harm the well being of a patient in the long run.

This work is aimed at providing the patients of epilepsy with an alternative treatment regimen. It would involve natural medicines instead of the allopathic ones. Minimal usage of chemicals is advocated, and the mode of proposed intervention is essentially non invasive.

Table of Contents

Table of Contents

A Proposed Psychophysical Exercise and Treatment Regimen for Epilepsy: Epilepsy Treatment by Therapeutic Aromatic Penetration and Olfactory Intervention (ETTAPOI)

Author: Arghya Ray

Date: January 2015

1. Introduction

The main issue with treating epilepsy is that epilepsy has several varieties. According to Tremblay (2015), localized epileptic disturbances may take place in primarily three parts of the brain. When the seizures take place in the temporal lobe, there are hallucinations involving a range of different senses such as vision, smelling, etc. For the purpose of this proposal, this type of epilepsy will be defined as variety 1 or V1 epilepsy. This is the most common type of epilepsy. Sometimes the seizures may take place in the occipital lobe, which create vision related problems. Only 5 to 10 percent of epilepsy cases fall in this category, and we will term it as variety 3 or V3 epilepsy. In the other category cases, which are more common than V3 but less common than V1, the frontal lobe is affected most. This kind of epilepsy results primarily into involuntary movements of muscles. We will term this category as V2.

The proposed therapeutic tool is to be defined as the Epilepsy Therapeutic Tool of Aromatic Penetration and Olfactory Intervention (ETTAPOI). This tool will be principally aimed at alleviating the sufferings due to V1 and V2 epileptic seizures. The tool is to be operated in coordination with the patient's act of breathing, and thereby, smelling. The sensory function of smelling is supposed to affect the coordination between different parts of the brain (see Frasnelli 2011). Nevertheless, the

ETTAPOI principally utilize the following postulate:

> If a sensory function is found to be excessively
> hyperactive or over-stimulated, then activate or
> stimulate at least one of its adjacent but less active
> or inactive sensory functions simultaneously.

Here, sensory function means activities like smelling a

flower, or watching a television, etc. The postulate can also

be tentatively applied to any real-world scenario related to

brain and nervous system.

2. Background Research

Although there is some scope of scholarly

argument, it is widely accepted that olfactory functioning

of brain is a very complex area of scientific exploration.

The complexity is mainly due to the fact that olfactory

functionality deeply embeds intra-brain coordination.

Unlike homeostasis (which is directly related with body

balancing), olfactory regions of brain serve the purpose of smelling but can affect across its various regions. As early as in the late 1980s, scientists like Cann and Ross (1989) were already exploring multidimensional associations between memory and smell. Cann and Ross (1989) conducted an experiment to show details of this presumed association. The experiment and results are concisely explained in the following paragraph:

"Olfactory stimuli were used as context cues in a recognition memory paradigm. Male college students were exposed to 50 slides of the faces of college females while in the presence of a pleasant or an unpleasant odor. During the acquisition phase, ratings of physical attractiveness of the slides were collected. After a 48-hr delay, a recognition test was given using the original 50 slides and 50 new slides. The recognition test was conducted with either the original odor or the alternative odor present. A no-odor control group did not receive olfactory cues.

The attractiveness ratings indicated that the odor

variations had no effect on these social judgments.

Analyses of d' scores, hits, and false alarms for the

recognition performance indicated support for the

predicted interaction in which presence of the same

odor at both sessions led to better overall

performance." (Cann and Ross 1989, p. 91)

Moreover, association between olfactory functions with a

particular sensory activity is also not atypical. Algom et al

(1993) established that odor and taste are highly

interrelated sensations that can be extensively utilized in

the field of psychophysics. Contextually, it should also be

mentioned that more recent research has detailed several

intra-brain coordination oriented functionalities and factors

with relation to olfactory activities and associated chemo-

sensations. In this milieu, according to Plailly et al (2008),

olfactory functions (and associated chemo-sensations) are

capable of affecting sensory coordination between the different parts of a human brain. These parts may include several regions of the brain spanning over mediodorsal thalamus, orbitofrontal cortex, neocortical projections, etc.

Furthermore, research done by Grabenhorst et al (2007) shows that the different parts of the olfactory regions of brain can be stimulated by different odors simultaneously. The authors also hint toward a possibility of olfactory activeness varying proportionally with the perceived degree of pleasantness (or unpleasantness) of the odor. As such, Grabenhorst et al (2007) also suggest that the olfactory regions like "orbitofrontal cortex and some connected regions represent separately the hedonically positive and the hedonically negative aspects of even a single stimulus such as an odor."

Last but not least, treatment by the means of stimulations is not unknown at all in the field of neuropsychiatry. Stimulation of motor cortex area, which is aimed at the treatment of neuropathic pain, has been reported by various researchers like Saitoh et al (2000), Radic et al (2015), etc. Nevertheless, there appears to be a chronic lack of research in the field of treatment by chemo-sensational methods. In this milieu, it is suggestible that strong smelling odors be utilized by the means of inhalation by the patient. As such, inhalation can be involuntary in the case the patient be kept in a controlled environment, and the odor be made strong enough with the help of concentrated amounts of suitable aromatic chemicals. Even unpleasant smells can be used depending on the patient response with an aim to incite chemo-sensation based activation of olfactory regions in the brain. With the help of academic correlation and previous research in this realm of neuroscience, it is already at least tentatively assumable that activation of different olfactory regions of the brain can lead to wider effects in the internal coordination of the brain tissues. Since major olfactory regions like the orbitofrontal cortex are embedded inside intricately networked neurons (crisscrossing all across various other parts of the brain), it is highly probable that controlled olfactory activations can lead to useful results at least for relatively shorter periods of time.

3. Proposed ETTAPOI Regimen

The theory of implementation is based on inhalation of odor by the patient. The ultimate goal is to achieve a "no seizures, no side effects" situation. In this context, inhalation of certain chemicals by the patient may prove to be beneficial for him/her.

3.1 Method of application

Sophisticated inhaling machinery must be used, where amount of the chemical can be controlled and odor quality can be tested when necessary. For example, an oxygen mask can be used. In the case the mask is used for supplying a smelling chemical, it can be termed as an aromatic mask designed especially for patients of epilepsy. Specific odors can be directed through the mask up to the nasal orifices of the patient.

3.2 Materials/chemicals to be used

Utilization of fuming aromatic compounds or smoke is potentially of no use given that the chemical being smelled is a stable, non-volatile compound. Instead, we would need a volatile chemical compound which would allow molecules to break away once subjected to suction. Volatile aromatic compounds with strong smell are suitable for this purpose since their physiochemical response to nasal suction is supposed to be very rapid.

3.3 Time of usage

Inhalation of the volatile chemical is to be done when the patient has an epileptic attack. In other words, a team of paramedical staffs or caregivers should be present at the time when the patient has seizures. And in serious cases, the aromatic mask will be used so that the patient, having seizures, involuntarily inhales the smell of the chemical to be administered.

3.4 For whom this intervention is meant

Patients suffering from V1, and particularly, V2 types of epilepsy are supposed to be benefited most. Patients who fail to smell or have other kinds of smelling problems (during seizures) may not be subjected to this regimen.

4. Tentative Flow of Intervention and Related Events

In this section, a list of bulleted points is given. These points are in a tentative sequence of events and interventions all during an epileptic attack.

- A patient is known to have either V1 or V2 type of epilepsy. Also, he/she does not have problems in smelling during seizures.

- The patient is kept under 24 hour's observation.

- As soon as the patient has seizure, he/she is to be first of all physically controlled by the caregivers. During the seizure, certain part or parts of the patient's brain are overactive, which needs to be controlled **(intervention step 1)**.

- Now an aromatic mask is positioned firmly over the nasal orifices of the patient suffering from seizure **(intervention step 2)**.

- ETTAPOI is based on balancing the overactive parts of the brain. It is supposed to prevent the asymmetric functioning of the brain (during seizures) by activating and/or stimulating the brain's different olfactory regions.

- The patient is allowed to grasp and inhale the odor. This odor will stimulate the olfactory regions and mitigate the existing asymmetric situation of the brain **(intervention step 3)**.

- Expected result is mitigation of the severity of the seizures in a gradual but faster fashion.

5. Proposed Aromatic Materials

An important point to be noted here is the terminological explanation of 'aromatic' or 'aroma.' With regard to ETTAPOI, the word aromatic does not mean just anything that smells. It denotes aromatic chemical compounds that have carbonaceous covalent bonding. In

ETTAPOI, the term aroma will generally denote the smell of an aromatic compound.

Before starting a discussion on what exact compounds can be utilized to create the necessary penetrative odor for ETTAPOI, it is necessary to find out how we should understand odor intensities with relation to the proposed treatment regimen. Jiang et al (2006) have made very useful contributions in the recent evolution of olfactometry. Accordingly, there are seven categories of perceived odor intensity or strength. These are tabulated below:

Table 1: Odor intensity evaluation scheme for aromatic compounds to be used in ETTAPOI. The scheme is adopted from Jiang et al (2006, p. 677).

Odor strength description	Odor intensity index/Equivalent feel of temperature
Extremely strong	6/ > 60°C
Very strong	5/ > 50°C
Strong	4/ > 40°C
Distinct	3/ > 30°C
Weak	2/
Very weak	1/
Non perceptible	0/

During the preliminary stages of intervention, the patient (in times of epileptic attack) should be subjected only to 'distinct' odors. That is to be produced by moderately concentrated aromatic vapors. If the patient is able to tolerate them without any significant side-effects or worsening of seizures, then the odor intensity is to be increased. Possibly, 'very strong' odors of aromatic compounds having medicinal value will prove to be suitable for later stages of intervention.

Another odor quality is to be considered which is not described in Jiang et al's (2006) odor intensity index development. It is the penetrative quality. Even strong odors like those of rotten eggs may not prove to be penetrative. Burrow et al (1983) have detected that the odors of camphor, menthol, etc. appear to have a penetrative property. Smelling them feels like clearance of the nasal pathways along with an effect of cold sensation. Penetrative properties of odors have yet not been measured, and they are chemo-sensational attributes that can possibly arouse psychophysical excitement and/or reaction in the patient.

Furthermore, in the light of previous research and well-known medicinal facts, two aromatic compounds appear to be highly suggestible for ETTAPOI use. Burrow et al's (1983) research is highly important from this perspective. Burrow et al (1983) have explained the medicinal value and chemo-sensational properties of eucalyptus, camphor, menthol, etc. For the purpose of ETTAPOI, we would first select camphor.

- Camphor is volatile

- Economic and generally available

- It has a penetrating smell

- The strong smell is thought to be capable of clearing nasal air passages

- Well-tolerated across a large number of individuals

- Capable of acting as an antidote to certain substances

Instead of focusing on the physiological and biomedical effects of inhaling camphor, it is important to focus on its chemo-sensational properties and capability of psychophysical influencing. According to Burrow et al (1983, p. 157):

> "Camphor, eucalyptus and menthol are traditionally believed to be of use in the symptomatic treatment of nasal congestion and their use in Otorhinolaryngology extends back over one hundred years."

Next, we would also suggest using citral. Citral is smells lemon-like, but the odor of this material is capable of qualifying as a penetrative odor. Citral already has medicinal and dietary value (Onawunmi 1989). There are certain benefits of using citral.

- Citral is less volatile than camphor, but yet it is considerably volatile.

- Economic and generally available

- A very small number of the population may have allergy to citral

- The strong smell is thought to be capable of clearing nasal air passages

Moreover, odor mixtures can also prove to be a winning option. Strong odors like those of petroleum, menthol, eucalyptus, gun powder, etc. can be artificially created or used with the help of respective raw substances. However, experimental testing is highly necessary, since ETTAPOI is a very novel regimen. Since the proposal-writer has not conducted any real world experiment or medical trial, the results remain completely unpredictable at this time. Although using compounds like camphor and citral can be winning options in the light of previous research, more improvisation will require extensive clinical trials. Before applying extraordinarily strong odors (those of petroleum, gun powder, etc.) on epileptic patients, sufficient number of clinical trial should also be conducted.

ETTAPOI, if implemented as a progressive treatment regimen, will indubitably result into controlled psychophysical exercise sessions. It is already known that mental exercises like memory game are helpful in refining or improving brain functions. Likewise, exercise of the neural networks inside one's brain can be beneficial in the long run. Olfactory intervention appears to be one of the best methods of conducting psychophysical exercise sessions. These sessions might also have a capability of causing considerable psychological refreshment and neurological rejuvenation of the patient. Furthermore, ETTAPOI can be used as a palliative measure that can have positive placebo effects as well.

6. Concluding Remarks

There are several risks associated with ETTAPOI. Firstly, there is a chronic lack in academic literature regarding research on nature of odors. There are no measurable parameters of how to detect a foul odor or distinguish a pleasant odor from an unpleasant one. For example, if Person A finds the smell of roses to be offensive but Person B finds the same smell to be pleasant, then we don't have any olfactometric method to understanding why two persons may have different opinions regarding the same odor. Secondly, the concept of penetrative odor is very important in implementing ETTAPOI. Researchers like Jiang et al (2006) have attempted to understand the various degrees of odor intensity. Yet, an intense odor may not be penetrative. For example, strong odor of ammonia cannot be placed in the same category of an equally intense odor of camphor. The substance to be used in ETTAPOI must have a strong plus penetrative odor. The property of penetration (which is a psychophysical feeling) can be well understood with the help of the works of Burrow et al (1983), where the authors have identified substances like camphor, eucalyptus, etc. having strong odor as well as nasal clearance or penetrative properties. However, research in this direction has not progressed much in the recent years. In sum, without a full knowledge of nature of odor and related olfactometric techniques readily available, ETTAPOI may not be as effective as it can be. As a result, it may even be discarded without the levels of scientific contemplation it deserves.

So, clinical trials among controlled groups should be carried out. Substances like camphor, citral, menthol, eucalyptus, etc. are already widely used. These aromatic substances can be utilized for implementing ETTAPOI in the beginning. Later on, clinicians may attempt to examine more substances having stronger odors. Before undergoing ETTAPOI, the participant or patient should also be tested for allergies, if any. Otherwise, the venture may become

too risky to carry out.

References

Algom, D., Marks, L. E., & Cain, W. S. (1993). Memory psychophysics for chemosensation: perceptual and mental mixtures of odor and taste. *Chemical Senses*, *18*(2), 151-160.

Burrow, A., Eccles, R., & Jones, A. S. (1983). The effects of camphor, eucalyptus and menthol vapour on nasal resistance to airflow and nasal sensation. *Acta oto-laryngologica*, *96*(1-2), 157-161.

Cann, A., & Ross, D. A. (1989). Olfactory stimuli as context cues in human memory. *The American journal of psychology*, 91-102.

Frasnelli, J. (2011). With which part of the brain do we smell? *Odotech*. Retrieved on 7th October 2015 from http://blog.odotech.com/part-brain-smell-special-guest-author-edition

Grabenhorst, F., Rolls, E. T., Margot, C., da Silva, M. A., & Velazco, M. I. (2007). How pleasant and unpleasant stimuli combine in different brain regions: odor mixtures. *The Journal of Neuroscience, 27*(49), 13532-13540.

Jiang, J., Coffey, P., & Toohey, B. (2006). Improvement of odor intensity measurement using dynamic olfactometry. *Journal of the Air & Waste Management Association, 56*(5), 675-683.

Onawunmi, G. O. (1989). Evaluation of the antimicrobial activity of citral.*Letters in applied microbiology, 9*(3), 105-108.

Plailly, J., Howard, J. D., Gitelman, D. R., & Gottfried, J. A. (2008). Attention to odor modulates thalamocortical connectivity in the human brain. *The Journal of Neuroscience, 28*(20), 5257-5267

Radic, J. A., Beauprie, I., Chiasson, P., Kiss, Z. H., &
Brownstone, R. M. (2015). Motor Cortex Stimulation for
Neuropathic Pain: A Randomized Cross-over
Trial. *Canadian Journal of Neurological Sciences/Journal
Canadien des Sciences Neurologiques*, 1-9.

Saitoh, Y., Shibata, M., Hirano, S. I., Hirata, M., Mashimo,
T., & Yoshimine, T. (2000). Motor cortex stimulation for
central pain and peripheral deafferentation pain: Report of
eight cases. *Journal of neurosurgery*, *92*(1), 150-155.

Tremblay, S. (2015). Different Parts of the Brain That
Epilepsy Effects, *Demand Media.* Retrieved on 7th October
2015 from http://www.livestrong.com/article/228934-
different-parts-of-the-brain-that-epilepsy-effects/

Notes

Notes

www.ingramcontent.com/pod-product-compliance
Lightning Source LLC
Chambersburg PA
CBHW061234180526
45170CB00003B/1296